YOUR KNOWLEDGE HAS VALUE

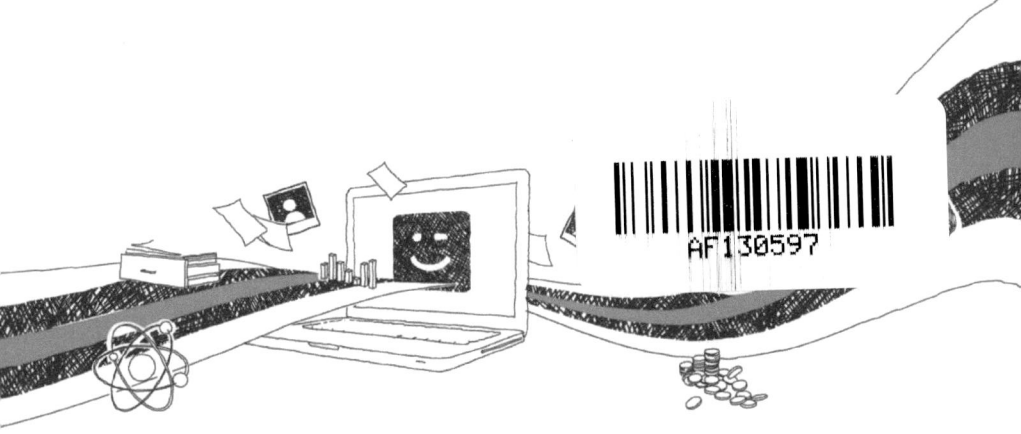

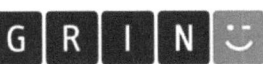

Breast Cancer Research. Ageing as Predisposing Factor

Gabby Ian

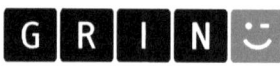

Bibliographic information published by the German National Library:

The German National Library lists this publication in the National Bibliography; detailed bibliographic data are available on the Internet at http://dnb.dnb.de.

ISBN: 9783346482822
This book is also available as an ebook.

Print and binding: Books on Demand GmbH, Norderstedt, Germany
Printed on acid-free paper from responsible sources.

The present work has been carefully prepared. Nevertheless, authors and publishers do not incur liability for the correctness of information, notes, links and advice as well as any printing errors.

GRIN web shop: https://www.grin.com/document/1045118

Ageing as Predisposing Factor for Breast Cancer

Contents

Abstract

This work investigates whether age is among the predisposing factors for breast cancer. Breast cancer is heterogeneous malignant cells whose specific age profiles exponentially increases until menopause after which it rises gently slowly thereby reflecting the superimposition of the early and late onset rates of breast cancer. The early onset breast cancers represents mainly the untimely life transforming or inherited consequences on the undeveloped epithelium, while late-onset breast cancers in most cases are likely to follow an extended exposure for supporting stimulus of vulnerable epithelium, which has botched to age normally. Biomarker studies and clinical observations indicates that the later staged breast cancer types often develop slowly and are less biologically aggressive compared to the early staged breast cancers despite being under the control of hormone receptors such as growth factor receptor abbreviated as (HER2) and estrogen receptor (ER), expressions hence supporting the conclusion that breast cancer biology is age dependent.

Approximately 12 percent of women across the globe in the current society are annually affected by breast cancer. Moreover, while breast cancer incidence increases with age advancement, patients of younger age at diagnosis are largely associated with increase in the mortality rate. This research discusses most of the age-related factors, which affect the identification or diagnosis, treatment, and management of breast cancer incidence; examining main concepts and exploring vital areas, which calls for additional research. Aging as a predisposing factor for breast cancer will be examined in connection to diagnosis and treatment with special reference to nodal status, hormone factors, breast cancer subtypes and genetic status.

Further, although narrowly, the study will also touch on the future expectations of breast cancer identification and treatment through examination of some of the rising potential technologies and breast cancer tests like the miRNA.

Introduction

Breast cancer is mainly the commonly diagnosed cancer disease among most women in the United Kingdom with the exclusion of squamous and basal cell carcinomas of the skin. It is foremost the leading cause of death for the majority of women globally, which accounts for about 22.5 percent of cancer incidences and 13 percent of all mortalities that are related to cancer. The lifetime risks of acquiring breast cancer, currently stand at 1 out of 8 women; however, more than 40 percent of the affected patients are 65 years and more, thus accounting for about 60 percent of the total deaths resulting from breast cancer incidences. It is interesting to note that the predisposing factor for developing breast cancer before 49 years is one out of fifty-three, which rises at 50-59 years to one out of forty-three and much higher between 60 and 69 years to one out of twenty-three (Torre et al., p, 103, 2015). Moreover, the risk of developing the disease increases significantly to 1/15 for women at 70 years and above.

Breast cancer mortality and incidence increase with age, hence it follows that older adults have a higher probability of developing breast cancer than younger adults and hence have high chances of dying of breast cancer. Elderly women, for instance, have about 3 times probability for breast cancer incidence compared to the younger population of 40 to 44 years of age and are 13 times on the mortality rate. According to the latest census conducted in the United Kingdom, there are more than 16 million Americans aged 75 years and above with 65 percent of the seniors being women. The risks of acquiring cancer greatly increase with age and the elderly are the fastest growing population segment in the UK. Research has established that this cancer of the breast is

4

the second most killer disease in women aged 75 and above years. This is particularly because of the risks of breast cancer nearly triple or doubles for women between 70 to 80 years of age at the rate of 23 in 500 women, compared to 8 in 500 women aged between 40 and 50 years (Torre et al., p, 103, 2015).

Despite taking several years of epidemiological research, and the identification of many risk factors influencing breast cancer, its occurrence has never been reduced so far. Although most medical practitioners continue to seek effective ways of preventing breast cancer, there have been indications of improvement in terms of early detection and treatment altogether, which have reduced the mortality rate of the disease. Research studies on the causes and effects of breast cancer have been on the progress to the point where currently, the cancer profile of a patient with higher risk of developing the disease can be described with some certainty. In this connection, people are gaining understanding and knowledge of the underlying biology concerning breast cancer including the molecular changes and hormonal influence, which contributes to its development and thrift (Bhaskaran et al., p, 561, 2014). The various scientific lines are converging to the suggestion that breast cancer occurs as a results of the combination of events and individual factors. These individual factors and events includes exposure to carcinogens for a longer period, inherited genetic vulnerability, variations in the molecular structure of DNA in breast cells, functions of the immune system of the body, and the levels of various hormones within the body among others. Moreover, nearly all of the recognized predisposing factors for breast cancer related to one or more of either the events or individual factors above.

Breast cancer occupies the first place categorically in women due to its high rates of mortality and incidence considering that it is hormone-related cancer whose occurrence is on the rise. The National Institute of Health and Medical Research estimates that the incidence of breast

5

cancer worldwide has doubled from 57 to 102 per 100,000 women between 1980 and 2005 mainly in developed countries such as the United Kingdom (Torre et al., p, 103, 2015). Breast cancer is one of the most significant public health problems considering that its diagnosis is usually delayed and its management is most often expensive and difficult to handle. According to research, the annual national cancer incidences were estimated at 36 000 new cancer cases with only 12,000 getting the required support. Nevertheless, this incidence has the shown the tendency of decreasing in the recent years because of the prevention tool which has proven effective in minimizing mortality from the disease often by stabilization of several risk factors and mammography screening.

Furthermore, breast cancer is a composite and clinically heterogeneous illness with several varied risk factors. Some of these risk factors responsible for its emergence include dietary and obesity factors, hormone replacement therapy for menopause, oral contraceptives, and exposure to ionization radiations. Family history of breast cancer, reproductive factors (such as not breastfeeding and late pregnancies), exogenous hormonal factors (like the hormone substitution treatment), endogenous hormonal factors (like late menopause and early age at menarche), and most specifically age are a few of the familiar risk factors for breast cancer incidence in most women. Although there has been high awareness level among both women and their physicians concerning the existence of these risk factors, the depth and magnitude of rising risks are usually not well understood. Age is, however, a very significant risk factor, which is often ignored. Although 1 in 8 women will eventually develop breast cancer with the estimate that women of 65 years and above faces the high risks of developing the disease (White et al., p, S9, 2014). The baseline level of risk for younger women is quite low and the chances of developing breast cancer from 35 to 55 years of age are only 2.5 percent, which is relevant particularly when

6

prophylactic mastectomy is put under consideration considering that this procedure will most likely be offered for younger women.

The total number of cases of elderly patients diagnosed with breast cancer is expected to increase swiftly in the future considering that over 15 percent of the current population is projected to rise above 65 years by 2030. In addition, improvements or advancements in the diagnosis and screening of the disease imply that the increasing population will have their breast cancer incidents detected quite at an early age. These anticipated trends together often result in a larger number of usually elderly patients who require management and lasting treatment of their breast cancer incidences. The acquisition of basic knowledge therefore on the mechanism of oncogenesis relating to the risk factors is an essential scientific direction for the development and improvement of current therapies and new therapeutic approaches. The objective and aim of this research study was to explore and analyze whether aging is among the predisposing factor for breast cancer for women in the United Kingdom. The consequences and impacts of modern investigations, findings and the available treatment options for the disease incidents will be examined in this study categorically by age bracket variation and how these variations affect changes in treatment options and further research.

Literature Review Related to the Topic

To begin with, cancer refers to an illness or condition where the abnormal cells begin to divide without invasion or control of the nearby tissues. Such cells are known as cancer cells, which may extend, to other parts of the body either via the blood system or through lymphatic systems (Torre et al., p, 89, 2015). Breast cancer on the other hand, is cancer, which emerges from the inner lining part of the milk lobules of the breast known as the lobular carcinoma. Cancer linked to breast very common invasive cancer type, which most often occurs in females worldwide.

AGING AS APREDISPOSING FACTOR FOR BREAST CANCER

A lot of women have been identified with breast cancer since 2004. At some point in this period, more than 2500 women died of breast cancer with the same disease accounting for more than 28,000 people losing their lives before reaching the age of 75 years. The rates of breast cancer incidence have been on the increase during the last two decades, whereas the mortality rates have been on the decline in the most recent decades. In approximation, half of the breast cancer cases affect women between 50 and 60 years. Furthermore, from the time when the national mammographic screening program was introduced in the United Kingdom, the incident rates for the disease have steeply increased for women between 50 and 69 years, which is the target group for the mammographic screening. It is most likely that increase in breast cancer incidence in the UK in the previous periods is largely because of the increased detection via the widespread application of mammographic screening (Chiarelli et al, p, 383, 2015).

Breast cancer affects both men and women; nevertheless, its rates of occurrence are much higher for women. Generally, women are at 100 fold higher probability of being diagnosed with breast cancer incident as compared to men since according to the research conducted in 2004 indicated that the standardized age incidents for breast cancer was one for every 100,000 men while for women, it was as high as 113 per 100,000 women (Torre et al., p, 103, 2015). Female sex can, therefore, be considered one of the major risk factors for this killer disease. Despite the major significant differences between men and women, being a woman is one of the strongest indicators that an ovarian and other female hormone plays an important task in the development and growth of breast cancer.

The incidence of breast cancer increases with age. Before the age of 25 years, it is a rare disease, however, its incidences increase steadily with age between 30 and 39 years and continue to increase gently to the oldest age. In the UK for instance, during early 2000, the incident rates of breast cancer was 5 for every 100,000 women between 20 and 29 years, which increased to 42 per 100,000 women between 30 to 39 years, 327 per 100,000 women during their 60s then rising steadily to 301 per 100,000 at 70 years and above . The reduction in the rate at which breast cancer rises around menopause further indicates that the ovarian and other active female hormones are responsible for breast cancer development (Copson et al., p, 983, 2013). On the contrary, the occurrence of other adult cancers, which are not hormone-dependent continuously, increases with age, with no indication of dampening during the mid-life. It is evident therefore that the increasing age and female sex are the two most probable risk factors for breast cancer. It follows therefore that the rate of incidence increase and decline during menopause are the indication that the ovarian and other female hormones contributes a significant role in the prevalence of breast cancer in women.

i. Lifetime Risks and Incidence of Breast Cancer by Age and Molecular Subtype

Breast cancer through molecular profiling has been grouped into four major subtypes, which are differentiated by their varying expression levels of the growth factor receptor- HER2, progesterone, and estrogen receptors which are represented by PR and ER respectively. These sub-branches include basal, HER2 Over-expressing, Lumina A, and Lamina B. Lamina type is the commonly prevalent breast cancer and is closely followed by HER2 Over-expression, then basal cancer (Maisonneuve et al., n.d, 2014). The below 40 years age bracket, perhaps unsurprisingly, is the majorly the most probable age group to present with the most aggressive or hostile triple-negative resistant subtype of breast cancer. Moreover, it is interesting to note that the same tendency continues up to 60 years of age, after which Lamina A takes the lead with the highest incident rate. It is most surprising, however, that Lamina A for under 50 years patients is the rarely common subtype of breast cancer despite being greatly influenced by minute proportions of breast

9

cancers subtypes prevalent in this age group (Maisonneuve et al., n.d, 2014). Triple negative, in the age bracket of between 50 and 59, is the most common subtype which is observed at 35 percent while Lamina A again is the least common subtype at about 28 percent, nevertheless, there are nearly equal chances of developing any subtype at this age bracket. In the 60-69 but less than 70s, age bracket as expected is that the most common breast cancer form is the Lamina subtype, which represents about 7 percent with triple-negative being the rarely prevalent subtype. Furthermore, Survival chances from breast cancer largely linked to the age at which the disease has been diagnosed considering that lesser survival rates is witnessed for patients with less than 50 years while for patients of 70 years and above have the least survival chances compared to those at their 50s.

Lamina A and Lamina B are the popular subtypes of breast cancer which have the tendencies of occurring in postmenopausal patients and most often have better outcomes compared to other subtypes (Maisonneuve et al., n.d, 2014). Moreover, these subtypes have been connected to the close contact with estrogen for nulliparous, however, those women undertaking hormone replacement therapy displays much higher risks. Because of this connection, anti-estrogen agents have been developed to limit the activities of estrogen by binding competitively the estrogen receptors (Davies et al., p, 811, 2013). According to Helvie et al, p, 2652, (2014), this treatment type is responsible for the improved disease-free endurance and the overall thrift in hormone-positive cancers, which includes 5 years of adjuvant tamoxifen management in the reduction of the yearly mortality by 31 percent across all age brackets.

ii. Genetics and Breast Cancer Risks with Age

Some of the genetic mutations that are of high-risk also affect the age of emergence and development. It has been established that 5.3 percent of breast cancer incidents for patients below 40 years are as a result of mutations in the Breast Cancer vulnerability gene 1 (BRCA1). This, however, decreases to 2.2 percent in the 40-49 age bracket and further drops to 1.1 percent for those developing breast cancers in the 50 to 70 years age group (Copson et al., p, 983, 2013). Moreover, it has been shown that patients having BRCA1l mutations have the high chances of developing basal-like cancers of the breast, which includes the molecular triple negative subtype.

BRCA1 and BRCA2 are presently the major genes, which influences breast cancer risks for patients depending on their age bracket. These genes act as tumor suppressor genes that are responsible for the repair of the damaged DNA and the mutation of these genes significantly leads to the amplified risk of breast cancer. Rough estimation indicates that about 16 percent of all familial breast cancer cases result from a mutation in these genes and contributes to about 5 percent of all breast cancer incidents. The probabilities of developing breast cancer for BRCA1 or BRCA2 mutation carriers stands at 57% and 49% respectively for those less than 70 years of age (Brohet et al., p, 102, 2014). It is worth noting that the BRCA mutation carriers often have the tendency of frequently developing more aggressive breast cancers at a tender age.

iii. Prognosis

Prognosis patients differ depending on their age variation. A younger woman will tend to have additional aggressive tumors like the triple negative types with a higher recurrence rate. The consequences are pronounced more for patients below 35 years of age. It has been confirmed that a tender age of diagnosis raises the mortality risk of breast cancer. These results because of lack of screening for women at a lower age, which implies that patients will often present bigger palpable lumps at advanced stages (Cappellani et al., n.d., 2013). Younger patients often have the tendencies of higher levels of Ki-67 (which are the indicators of poor prognostic outcome) with the highest level witnessed for patients less than 35 years of age (Gallardo & Lerma, p, 1, 2017). Nevertheless, some recent studies contradict that the mortality rates are in no way associated with the age differences mainly because of the improved treatment options, early identification of high-risk patients, and the current advances in screening. Recent studies have further shown that women of 55 years old and above have a better prognosis with similar survival to the general population regardless of the disease status. By reflecting on the younger patients, women at the end of the age spectrum of less than 70 years also present with the advanced tumors.

Several patients in the past were deemed unsuitable for medical surgery due to their age and medical co-morbidities like chronic gastritis, asthma, stroke, hypertension, coronary heart disease, and diabetes mellitus among others. These co-morbidities act as independent risk factors for survival and are found disproportionally in older patients. The improved surgical method implies that a larger percentage of these patients can now successfully undergo curative surgeries for their conditions. These conditions can further provide makers for assessing chemotherapy suitability in connection with the established factors like the comprehensive geriatric assessment (CGA). Recent studies have established that frailty and malnutrition are the biggest risk factors for mortality in patients with breast cancer particularly those above 70 years of age. A CGA is capable of providing relevant age-related information that indicates which patients would be fit for chemotherapy treatment (Königsberg et al., p, 200, 2016). HER2 breast cancer types, on the other hand, are characterized by the over-expression of HER2 that is a high-grade tumor in general. These often have the tendencies of growing rapidly considering that, they are associated with relatively poor prognosis, nevertheless, they usually respond to treatment with the Herceptin (trastuzumab). HER2 breast cancer subtypes are usually classified further depending on their expression of lack of expression of ER

iv. The length of menstrual cycle and the Age at menarche

Menarche, which is the time of menstrual cycles, is often characterized by cellular proliferation in the breast, ovulation, and monthly fluctuations in hormone levels. In reality, the breast commences its growth 1-2 years prior to menarche, and this growth of the breast tissues is witnessed during the period of early adolescence. The breast epithelial cells in this immature state are considered vulnerable to random errors and carcinogens in the genetic material, which can be passed on to other additional breast cells as they divide. Age at thelarche, which is the age of breast development and the age at menarche have progressively, decreased in various parts of the globe during the last century. Factors that are responsible for the decrease in the age at menarche includes an increase in body size, improved nutrition, and the attainment of enough body fats to start the reproductive life. The increase in the body mass index (BMI) and height are said to accelerate the onset of menarche most probably because it depends on the attainment of the critical body mass (Rosner et al., 2009, 2017). In the early centuries before 1950, the age at menarche fell by 2-3 per calendar decade in the USA and UK, the decline that has been associated with the increase in the incidences of breast cancer.

The epidemiological research studies of breast cancer have indicated that women who experienced their initial menstrual periods at less than 12 years of age slightly have higher risks of breast cancer of 10 to 25 percent compared to women who had their menstrual periods in the later years of 12 years and above. This is true particularly because early menarche prolongs the exposure of a woman to oestrogens and other female hormones that are responsible for breast cancer. Studies have further indicated that women experiencing an early age at menarche have the most probability of higher oestrogens for much longer years after menarche, which might extend to their entire reproductive lives, which is not the case for women with late menarche (Pascual et al., p, 21943, 2017). Early menarche is also said to be connected with regular ovulatory cycles, which contributes to significant lifetime exposure of the breast tissues to the endogenous hormones. Shorter length cycles have been further shown to increase the risks for breast cancer in women. This is attributed particularly to the frequent cycles and the much time spent in the luteal phase, the period when progesterone and estrogen levels are high and the cell proliferation in the breast tissues appears higher.

Younger age for parous women is associated with lower lifetime risks for breast cancer at first childbirth. However, a collaborative data analysis restricted to women with no breastfeeding history indicates that the relative risks for breast cancer decrease at 3 percent every year younger from the age at which the first child was born (Biesaga et al., p, 7648, 2016). The women who have their first child at a younger age of below 25 years have a breast cancer risk of about 43 percent which is lower compared to the risks for women who have their first child at a later age of 29 years and above, irrespective of the duration of breastfeeding and the number of children. However, for some women who have their first child at 29 years and above, particularly those who had one child and never breastfed them have a higher breast cancer risks compared to nulliparous women. Further evidence suggests that the increased risks associated with late first birth age are stronger for premenopausal cancer compared to the postmenopausal breast cancer.

v. Age at Menopause

During, menopause, a process called involution in addition to the gradual cessation of ovarian hormone production occurs in the breast; this process is characterized by the reduction in the proliferation cell and an ultimate decrease in the proportion of epithelial cells. The postmenopausal women have between 15 and 50 percent lower breast cancer risk compared to premenopausal women of the same age and childbearing. The risks for acquiring breast cancer for postmenopausal women is lower compared to premenopausal women, it, however, increases with age at menopause. The risks for breast cancer is lower for the women who experience menopause at 40 years and below, while for late menopause women, the risk is close to those of premenopausal women of the same age at 55 years and above. Women of 55 years and above at menopause have twice the risk of breast cancer compared to women at 45 years who experience natural menopause (Biesaga et al., p, 7648, 2016).

vi. microRNAs and breast cancer

Recently, age has been implicated as a factor influencing the varied expressions of microRNA (miRNA) which are 19-25 long non-protein RNA coding, which is involved in the apoptosis, proliferation, cell differentiation, and development. More than 2000 different miRNAs have been currently recognized in humans where they regulate an estimate of 30 percent of all human genes. The current research that has been focused on the task of breast cancer in relation to miRNAs implicates the abnormal miRNA guideline as a factor in breast cancer introduction and development. Further research on the consequences of age on breast cancer incidences, and the circulating miRNA may increase additional insights into the identification, variation or the available treatment options available for breast cancer patients for every distinct age group.

With the ever-intensifying knowledge of breast cancer and its age-related consequences, there have been gradual improvements in the guiding principle concerning treatment and other best practices. Detection and survival rates over the last few decades have improved immensely despite the absence of consensus in the management of the younger population of below 35 years and the increasingly elderly population of over 70 years. An improved knowledge and understanding of the breast cancer genetics via molecular profiling are capable of providing valuable information, which can be applied, to both the young and old patients. This concept has been verified through the discovery of the high-risk BRCA genes, which provides a very crucial explanation to younger patients regarding their breast cancer conditions. There are however no clear guiding principle for the care and management of breast cancer patients above 65 years of age (Helvie et al., p, 2452, 2015). Moreover, scoring systems such as miRNA or CGA profiles are capable of providing accurate ways to determine which patients are to receive palliative or active treatments. Nevertheless, advance investigations are needed to determine the practicality and feasibility of such systems, which can further steps towards personalized treatment plans for breast cancer disease.

The larger majority of individual malignancies are age-connected cancers, which indicates incidence rates which increases exponentially with age throughout old age such that a larger percentage of all invasive cancers occurs among the vulnerable population of 55 years and above. Cancer incidences in the United Kingdom have been under monitory for a long time by the End Results from the program of the National Cancer Institute, Epidemiology, and Surveillance, which collects data from various registries across the state representing about 26 percent of the total population. About 80 percent of all breast cancer cases arise in women at the age of 50 years or older and rises from below 1.5 percent the probability of increasing invasive percent at 40 years to approximately 3 percent at 50 years, and 4 percent at 70 years; this produces, therefore, a lifetime risk of 1 in 8 breast cancer cases for women.

While aging is highly personalized, the standard age-associated changes represent a constantly changing tissue conditions from where malignancy should be differentiated. A number of the normal specific organ aging may constitute reduced tissue function or mass such as skeletal muscles, kidney, and liver among others; loss of functional reserve without significant loss of tissue mass, or tissue to remold the altered organ function (Olsson et al., p, 229, 2013). For nulliparous women (women who are not pregnant and have never have children), the ovarian size and function reduce progressively after the second decade of life. They further losses their breast glandular mass progressively which are then replaced by the combination of the college nous stoma and fatty tissues.

The cellular and molecular impacts of normal aging compared to those of natural menopause are the ovarian estrogen production, which in turn affects the ER expressing organ such as the breast. The ER expression in the ordinary breast indicates a measured >3 fold rise in the start of the third decade and further plateauing by the sixth life decade. However, the estrogen-inducible protein such as PR does not indicate any important specific age change in their median level of expression in the ordinary breast, despite being subjected to variations within every menstrual cycle. More complicated age-related impacts on the typical mammary glands are the variable but marked age connected the rise in the breast stromal and adipose cell production of aromatase, enzyme that is prearranged by the *CYP19A1* gene (Early Breast Cancer Trialists' Collaborative Group, p, 1347, 2015). The testosterone and androstenedione whose levels of serum in the postmenopausal women is not much decrease from the ones present in the follicular phase premenopausal women are the precursors that are androgenic in nature converted by aromatase into estradiol (E2) and estrone (Giusti et al., p, 37, 2011). Therefore it follows that the age-related amplification in mammary gland aromatase production is in a way that the levels of the mammary glands are able to approach those of the premenopausal mammary glands.

Furthermore, age as a marker of time captures the duration of accumulation and exposure to cancer risks. In this connection, nine hallmarks of aging have been proposed and they include epigenetic alteration and instability, which also marks the hull marks for breast cancer. Several studies have proved that the relationships between breast cancer and age are due fundamentally to the time accumulation of epigenetic and genetic mutations and to the increased susceptibility of the adults to the oncogenic mutations. The multifactorial transformation process from normal cells to breast cancer involves the accumulation of the DNA damage and mutation for a specific period catalyzed with the disruptions of the DNA repair and the system of cell growth regulation (Lodi et al., p, 4,9, 2014).

Health at midlife lays the foundation for longevity and health at a later stage in life. This is also the period in which most well-recognized risk factors for breast cancer and other diseases begins to show impacts. Moreover, the prevalence of various preventable diseases and chronic conditions like diabetes and obesity shows the tendency of increasing during midlife, and these conditions have demonstrated strong connections with increased breast cancer risks and minimal cancer survival rates. Despite the perception that the members of the current generation of adults of 45 to 64 years are expected to live longer compared to earlier generation members, they face the higher rates of chronic conditions, which are major risk factors for breast cancer compared to the previous generation. Promotion of general health through exercises and other means and the Prevention or management of these chronic conditions during midlife, therefore, are promising strategies for preventing or delaying breast cancer incidences at older ages.

In 2002, more than 40,000 cancer registrations in the UK were attributed to breast cancer. Save for being a female gender, the most fundamental factor for breast cancer is the rising age, which we have no control of. It is of great importance, therefore; when a woman acknowledges that the risk of breast cancer increases with age considering that their knowledge on the increased risks will help them inform their health-seeking behavior (Hanahan & Weinberg, p,

469, 2011). Furthermore, a delay or prevention of a cancer occurrence in an individual can be seen as an effective strategy for attaining a long and healthier life. Hence, by application of the presently available scientific evidence, we can be able to promote cancer prevention at midlife since it will be possible to significantly modify the relationship between age and breast cancer risks.

Methodology

The study was Biological-based where various previous studies and researches were thoroughly analyzed to identify whether age is among the predisposing factors responsible for breast cancer incidence among women in the United Kingdom. Various studies were retrieved from various library databases, which include the, UK cancer research database, Haden Madden Library database, Winley online portal among others with the same contents regarding risk factors associated with breast cancer. Data found within these the databases and various journals proved detrimental in understanding the connection between age and breast cancer incidences. The study was not only focused on the connection between age as a risk factor but also to other age-related effects of the breast cancer in relation to other risk factors responsible for breast cancer emergence. This was particularly essential considering that the various case studies presented were able to show data that were used to compare and contrast cancer effects among different age groups.

Case 1: A Meta-analysis and Systematic Review of the Risk Factors for Breast Cancer for Women of between 40 and 60 Years

A standard protocol to be followed was developed for this review. The researchers in conjunction with the research librarian made use of the Database of Systematic Reviews, Central Register of Controlled Trials and the National Library of Medicine and Medical Subject Heading for relevant systematic reviews on the aging as a predisposing factor for breast cancer. The researchers conducted secondary referencing through manual review of the reference lists including reviewing of the citations of fundamental studies by the application of the Scopus. Searched included studies of publications within the past 16 years, which they perceived, could provide relevant data on the current women cohorts with the consideration of mammography screening. This was to correspond to the timeframe data for age risk factor collected by the Breast cancer surveillance consortium for the study.

The researchers developed an exclusion and inclusion technique for articles and abstracts based on the outcome measures, risk factors, and the target population under consideration. They included meta-analyses, systematic reviews, observational studies, and randomized controlled trials. After the initial abstract reviews, full-text articles were retrieved for the second review by the application of the additional inclusion criteria specifically designed for each risk factor, which included the eligibility of the statistical data meta-analysis. The target population for the research mainly consisted women between 40 and 60 years of age and who were eligible for mammography screening.

Case 2: A Vivid Analysis of the Progesterone Receptor Negative, Estrogen Receptor Negative, and HER2 Negative Invasive Breast Cancers or rather the Triple Negative Phenotypes

In this case study, researchers identified and examined patients with triple negative breast cancers of varied age groups by the application of the UK Cancer Registry data between 1999 and 2003. The total number of women diagnosed with the primary breast cancer was 92,358, out of which 53.3% (51,074) had the three makers with only 6370 being considered triple negative breast cancer cases. The rest of the populations were however considered any other types of breast cancer.

The researchers managed to use the cases in the comparison of triple negative breast cancers among patients of various age groups, which was further based on their relative survival and social economic status.

The cases ware identified categorically by the use of medical records. In identifying whether the cases were triple negative breast cancers, HER2, PR, and ER receptors would be negative (absent). PR and ER receptors are found to be negative if the immunoperoxidase staining of a tumor cell nucleus was below 5 percent (Katrina, n.d., 2007). The pathologists, in this case, applied the immunohistochemistry technique where the results are on a qualitative scale ranging from 0 to 3+ to determine whether HER2 is negative for different age group patients if the results were 0 and 1+. Moreover, medical results were applied in the identification of whether age, relative survival, and socioeconomic conditions were risk factors for breast cancer. The case was conducted among different age group patients from different ethnic backgrounds and environments.

Results

From the Cancer Research Database in the UK, it was established that some of the things, which increases the risk of breast cancer, included certain medical conditions, hormone levels, lifestyle factors, and most specifically Age among others. From the Website, it was clear that breast cancer is the most common cancer type in the United Kingdom with the exclusion of the nonmelanoma skin cancer and is the most common cancer type affection quite a number of women in the UK. It followed that 1 in 870 men and 1 in 8 women in the UK had the record of breast cancer during their lifetime. On the risk factors responsible for breast cancer, it was evident that most breast cancer incidences occur in women above 50 years and was very rare for women below 40 years. Further, it was clear that in order to pick up cancer early, having mammograms as part of the national breast screening programmed was very fundamental. The portal, therefore, indicated that all women aged between 50 and 70 were open for the invitation for screening by the UK screening programme (Marmot et al., p, 2205, 2013). These were in the efforts to take control of breast cancer, which was rated the second most killer disease in the country.

Results from case 1 indicated that age is among the predisposing factors for breast cancer incidences among women across the globe. It was established that breast cancer was prevalence at an advanced age compared to younger adults of less than 40 years. However, the delayed presentation of symptomatic breast cancer has the most probability for the younger women globally across the various ethnic divide. Older women despite being at a higher probability of developing breast cancer compared to younger women, they are in particular poor at identifying other predisposing factors and symptoms of breast cancer. Nevertheless, the age controversy was indicated in some of the reviewed journals considering that there was variation in the exact age brackets in which breast cancer is prevalent in a particular age bracket. About 20 percent demonstrated that age does not matter with some advocating for 80 years as the most risk age for breast cancer incidence (McGuire et at., p, 822, 2015). The study also established that there exist various subtypes of breast cancer women, which are also clustered among different patients depending on their age groups. Further, it was evident that certain molecular and cellular reactions and variations depending on age also contribute to breast cancer menace among women; these entailed the various reproductive health variations among different women worldwide with regard to their age brackets.

From case2, based on the analysis, the majority of the women with triple-negative breast cancer were found mostly at more advanced stages in comparison to other groups. Patients who were 40 years and below were 1.53 times likely to have the triple negative breast cancer compared to those aged around 60 years and above (Go, Chung, & Park, p, 1284, 2016). The study demonstrated that the women with triple negative cancer only had 77 percent chances for survival five years from diagnosis compared to those who had other breast cancer types at 93 percent.

Discussion

Elderly women will continue to represent an increased fraction of the total number of women diagnosed with breast cancer as the population ages. By application of data from the large population-based cohort, it has been established that family history and most specifical age at menopause continue to influence the risk of breast cancer among women of 75 years and above. A modifiable risk factor for high body mass index was consistently connected with the rise in breast cancer risk for every age group in this postmenopausal cohort of women (Lauby-Secretan et al., p, 2355, 2015). It has been established that higher proportions with favorable characteristics such as histology's, which are tumors that are neither lobular nor ductal, positive estrogen receptor, and local stage at diagnosis characterized breast cancer occurring in elderly women of 75 years and above at diagnosis.

The existing literature on the risk factors for breast cancer indicates that age heterogeneity is the most evident after putting into consideration the role of body fatness, which is often measured by the body mass index. Several studies have revealed that the relationship between breast cancer and high body mass index is null and inverse upon the consideration of cancer diagnosed prior to menopause, however high body mass index is associated with the rise in the breast cancer risk for postmenopausal women. Prior studies, which considered the contributions of the high body mass index by age group among postmenopausal women largely, suggested that relative breast cancer risk factors were stronger in the elderly age bracket. For instance, part of the study on the odds ratio for the lowest versus highest quintile of body mass index rose from 1.5 for women diagnosed between 60 and 69 years to 2.8 for those aged 70 years and above at diagnosis (Kunkler et al., p, 271, 2015).

An early age at first live birth and the increased number of births are considered as protective against postmenopausal breast cancer. The available data indicates that a high number of births among parous women is associated with the reduction in the risk for breast cancer on all age groups of postmenopausal women, which includes those aged 75, and above years. It was established that age and null parity at first live birth had little connection with breast cancer for the elderly women. From the patient population under consideration, the most common treatment form for breast cancer was surgery, which can be breast-conserving surgery or mastectomy (Boyd et al, p, 417, 2014). A good number of operations were performed successfully with some women undergoing multiple procedures. It was observed that the most common of adjuvant treatment was the hormonal therapy that was given to about 70 percent of women. The characteristics or behavior of primary tumors in older women are homogenous considering that more than 60 percent were PR positive while more than 75 percent were ER-positive and only a few were HER2/ neu positive.

Like many common cancers, breast cancer is a disease primarily for older adults, particularly elderly women. In the United Kingdom, the average age at the diagnosis of breast cancer is 60 years and about 40 percent of breast cancers are diagnosed in women of 65 years and above. The average age of most death occurrences from breast cancer is 68 years with about 57 percent of breast cancer deaths occurring in those with 65 years and above. Breast cancer at the early stages for both younger and older adults are curable in a good number of patients since over 1 million elderly women in the UK are breast cancer survivors and above 800,000 of them are 75 years and above (Ayvaci et al., p 584, 2014). Breast cancer mortality and incidence increase with age, hence it follows that older adults are likely to develop breast cancer than younger adults and hence are more likely to die of breast cancer. Elderly women, for instance, have about 3 times probability for breast cancer incidence compared to the younger population of 40 to 44 years of age and are 13 times on the mortality rate.

According to the latest census conducted in the United Kingdom, there are more than 16 million Americans aged 75 years and above with 65 percent of the seniors being women. The risks of acquiring cancer greatly increase with age and the elderly are the fastest growing population segment in the UK. Research has established that cancer is the second most killer disease in women aged 75 years and above. This is particularly because of the risks of breast cancer nearly triple or doubles for women between 70 to 80 years of age at the rate of 23 in 500 women, compared to 8 in 500 women aged between 40 and 50 years (Moss et al., p, 1226, 2015). It was unfortunate however that, patients above 65 years particularly those over 80 are usually underrepresented in clinical trials and are either not enrolled or overtly excluded.

There has never been a standard care, which has been agreed upon to care for elderly women with breast cancer. Moreover, the screening guidelines for annual mammograms are contradictory and vague to certain limits. It follows then that the decision to continue with breast cancer screening for elderly women is a very controversial issue, and the quest for treatment for freshly discovered breast cancers in these women is similarly a fundamental decision, which lacks data. Factors influencing treatment pattern are difficult to measure and report, however, the patients in most cases make use of their own psychological factors and the physician recommendation, which are the most influential factors when making decisions pertaining treatment (Ory et al., p, s4. 2014). The healthcare providers often may not recommend treatment given the heterogeneity of the population despite the availability of evidence that octogenarian women with breast cancer die from their disease usually as younger women (Liu et al., p, 881,

2016). Moreover, evidence indicates that older women on most occasions tend to face the similar under goings as younger women with comparable treatment.

Limitations

This study was applied as a structured approach to literature review; nevertheless, there was some inherent limitation to the approach. One of the major challenges is that systematic reviews are often limited by the quality and quantity of the studies to be included in the review and the methodology to be applied. The research has been having been limited through the restriction to the English language. Language restrictions in most cases tend to result in study biases whose direction cannot be determined. The research study has been further limited to the published academic literature, which includes journals, and peer reviews thereby disregarding most of the unpublished literature work concerning the search topic. This restriction to the published literature is most probably likely to lead to some form of biased considering that most of the unpublished work present on the research topic of aging and breast cancer consists of studies, which do not necessarily identify or focus on significant results.

Moreover, the research varied by reference groups, measures, and the adjustments for cofounders which results in multiple risks of factors not being considered. The research was also limited to the establishment whether aging was a risk factor for breast cancer, hence while conducting the research, other prevalent risk factors had to be ignored despite others having a special connection with age effect on breast cancer incidence. Hence, it was quite a task in selecting an appropriate article, journal, or website among others that were solely based on aging as a predisposing factor for breast cancer. This was particularly hectic part considering the research was qualitative and relied on the available reference materials, which in most instances gave a detailed description of general risk factors for breast cancer.

Conclusion

In conclusion, breast cancer is much prevalent in older people compared to younger ones mainly because of their prolonged exposure to carcinogens such as environmental chemicals, radiation, sunlight, and substances present in the food taken. Mutation is also believed to occur due to the random errors when the DNA cells are copied before their division hence our cells accumulate more mutations as the age increases. Moreover, changes in the organs and tissues with the advancing age renders the microenvironment for the cells more favorable for the development of breast cancer in older people. People are therefore required to understand that if breast cancer is detected earlier, then thousands of lives can be saved yearly (Webber et al., n.d., 2017). Furthermore, it is particularly advisable for one to seek assistance from health care practitioners as well as take advantage of the available screening tests to minimize the risk of developing cancer of the breast. If an individual chooses to undertake cancer screening, he or she has a greater chance of extending their lifespan and it has a positive health implication. It is also essential for health care practitioners to offer evocative counseling about cancer of the breast. The counseling should collectively progress from both outside sources and personal experience to elevate the alertness of early breast cancer detection via proper methods of screening.

Recommendations

Since breast cancer is age dependent as have been demonstrated, it follows that people should take precautions against other risk factors that support breast cancer incidence by heeding to the following recommendations:

(a).   Women ought to desist from drinking alcoholic beverages completely to reduce the risk of developing breast cancer.

(b).   Women should be encouraged partake in at least some weekly exercises to minimize the risk of developing cancer of the breast.

(c).   Post-menopausal hormone therapy should be limited to minimize the risk that is linked to development of breast cancer

(d).   Females who frequently breastfeed often are at a lesser risk of developing breast cancer compared to those who do not. Therefore, women should be encouraged to breastfeed frequently.

(e).   Further comprehensive research should be conducted on the incorporation of both 2D and 3D mammography to ensure their precision and accuracy in detection of breast cancer so that they can be used on humans.

Bibliography

Ayvaci, M.U., Alagoz, O., Chhatwal, J., del Rio, A.M., Sickles, E.A., Nassif, H., Kerlikowske, K. and Burnside, E.S., 2014. Predicting invasive breast cancer versus DCIS in different age groups. BMC cancer, 14(1), p.584.

Bhaskaran, K., Douglas, I., Forbes, H., dos-Santos-Silva, I., Leon, D.A. and Smeeth, L., 2014. Body-mass index and risk of 22 specific cancers: a population-based cohort study of 5• 24 million UK adults. The Lancet, 384(9945), pp.755-765.

Biesaga, B., Niemiec, J., Wysocka, J., Słonina, D. and Ziobro, M., 2016. The search for optimal cutoff points for apoptosis and proliferation rate in prognostification of early-stage breast cancer patients treated with anthracyclines in adjuvant settings. Tumor Biology, 37(6), pp.7645-7655.

Boyd, N.F., Huszti, E., Melnichouk, O., Martin, L.J., Hislop, G., Chiarelli, A., Yaffe, M.J. and Minkin, S., 2014. Mammographic features associated with interval breast cancers in screening programs. Breast Cancer Research, 16(4), p.417.

Brohet, R.M., Velthuizen, M.E., Hogervorst, F.B., Meijers-Heijboer, H.E., Seynaeve, C., Collée, M.J., Verhoef, S., Ausems, M.G., Hoogerbrugge, N., van Asperen, C.J. and García, E.G., 2014. Breast and ovarian cancer risks in a large series of clinically ascertained families with a high proportion of BRCA1 and BRCA2 Dutch founder mutations. Journal of medical genetics, 51(2), pp.98-107.

Cappellani, A., Di Vita, M., Zanghì, A., Cavallaro, A., Piccolo, G., Majorana, M., Barbera, G. and Berretta, M., 2013. Prognostic factors in elderly patients with breast cancer. BMC Surgery, 13(2), p.S2.

AGING AS APREDISPOSING FACTOR FOR BREAST CANCER

Chiarelli, A.M., Prummel, M.V., Muradali, D., Shumak, R.S., Majpruz, V., Brown, P., Jiang, H., Done, S.J. and Yaffe, M.J., 2015. Digital versus screen-film mammography: impact of mammographic density and hormone therapy on breast cancer detection. Breast cancer research and treatment, 154(2), pp.377-387.

Copson, E., Eccles, B., Maishman, T., Gerty, S., Stanton, L., Cutress, R.I., Altman, D.G., Durcan, L., Simmonds, P., Lawrence, G. and Jones, L., 2013. Prospective observational study of breast cancer treatment outcomes for UK women aged 18–40 years at diagnosis: the POSH study. Journal of the national cancer institute, 105(13), pp.978-988.

Davies, C., Pan, H., Godwin, J., Gray, R., Arriagada, R., Raina, V., Abraham, M., Alencar, V.H.M., Badran, A., Bonfill, X. and Bradbury, J., 2013. Long-term effects of continuing adjuvant tamoxifen to 10 years versus stopping at 5 years after diagnosis of estrogen receptor-positive breast cancer: ATLAS, a randomised trial. The Lancet, 381(9869), pp.805-816.

Early Breast Cancer Trialists' Collaborative Group, 2015. Aromatase inhibitors versus tamoxifen in early breast cancer: patient-level meta-analysis of the randomised trials. The Lancet, 386(10001), pp.1341-1352.

Gallardo, A. and Lerma, E., 2017. Response letter to Questions about Ki67 staining in luminal breast cancer. Breast Cancer Research and Treatment, pp.1-1.

Giusti, F., Ottanelli, S., Masi, L., Amedei, A., Brandi, M.L. and Falchetti, A., 2011. Construction of a database for the evaluation and the clinical management of patients with breast cancer treated with antiestrogens and/or aromatase inhibitors. Clinical cases in mineral and bone metabolism, 8(1), p.37.

Go, Y., Chung, M., and Park, Y., 2016. Dietary Patterns for Women With Triple-negative Breast Cancer and Dense Breasts. Nutrition and cancer, 68(8), pp.1281-1288.

Hanahan, D. and Weinberg, R.A., 2011. Hallmarks of cancer: the next generation. cell, 144(5), pp.646-674.

Helvie, M.A., Chang, J.T., Hendrick, R.E. and Banerjee, M., 2014. Reduction in late-stage breast cancer incidence in the mammography era: Implications for overdiagnosis of invasive cancer. Cancer, 120(17), pp.2649-2656.

Helvie, M.A., Chang, J.T., Hendrick, R.E. and Banerjee, M., 2014. Reduction in late-stage breast cancer incidence in the mammography era: Implications for overdiagnosis of invasive cancer. Cancer, 120(17), pp.2649-2656.

Katrina, K.B. (2007). Descriptive Analysis of Estrogen Receptor Negative, Progesterone

Receptor Negative, and HER2-Negative Invasive Breast Cancer, the So-called

Triple-Negative Phenotype. Cancer

Königsberg, R., Pfeiler, G., Hammerschmid, N., Holub, O., Glössmann, K., Larcher-Senn, J. and Dittrich, C., 2016. Breast Cancer Subtypes in Patients Aged 70 Years and Older. Cancer Investigation, 34(5), pp.197-204.

Kunkler, I.H., Williams, L.J., Jack, W.J., Cameron, D.A. and Dixon, J.M., 2015. Breast-conserving surgery with or without irradiation in women aged 65 years or older with early breast cancer (PRIME II): a randomised controlled trial. The lancet oncology, 16(3), pp.266-273.

Lauby-Secretan, B., Scoccianti, C., Loomis, D., Benbrahim-Tallaa, L., Bouvard, V., Bianchini, F. and Straif, K., 2015. Breast-cancer screening—viewpoint of the IARC Working Group. New England Journal of Medicine, 372(24), pp.2353-2358.

Liu, B., Floyd, S., Pirie, K., Green, J., Peto, R., Beral, V. and Million Women Study Collaborators, 2016. Does happiness itself directly affect mortality? The prospective UK Million Women Study. The Lancet, 387(10021), pp.874-881.

Lodi, M., Scheer, L., Reix, N., Heitz, D., Carin, A.J., Thiébaut, N., Neuberger, K., Tomasetto, C. and Mathelin, C., 2017. Breast cancer in elderly women and altered clinicopathological characteristics: a systematic review. Breast Cancer Research and Treatment, pp.1-12.

Maisonneuve, P., Disalvatore, D., Rotmensz, N., Curigliano, G., Colleoni, M., Dellapasqua, S., Pruneri, G., Mastropasqua, M.G., Luini, A., Bassi, F. and Pagani, G., 2014. Proposed new clinicopathological surrogate definitions of luminal A and luminal B (HER2-negative) intrinsic breast cancer subtypes. Breast Cancer Research, 16(3), p.R65.

Marmot, M.G., Altman, D.G., Cameron, D.A., Dewar, J.A., Thompson, S.G., Wilcox, M. and Independent UK Panel on Breast Cancer Screening, 2013. The benefits and harms of breast cancer screening: an independent review: A report jointly commissioned by Cancer Research UK and the Department of Health (England) October 2012. British journal of cancer, 108(11), p.2205.

McGuire, A., Brown, J.A., Malone, C., McLaughlin, R., and Kerin, M.J., 2015. Effects of age on the detection and management of breast cancer. Cancers, 7(2), pp.908-929.

Moss, S.M., Wale, C., Smith, R., Evans, A., Cuckle, H. and Duffy, S.W., 2015. Effect of mammographic screening from age 40 years on breast cancer mortality in the UK Age trial at 17 years' follow-up: a randomised controlled trial. The Lancet Oncology, 16(9), pp.1123-1132.

Olsson, Å., Sartor, H., Borgquist, S., Zackrisson, S. and Manjer, J., 2014. Breast density and mode of detection in relation to breast cancer-specific survival: a cohort study. BMC cancer, 14(1), p.229.

Ory, M.G., Anderson, L.A., Friedman, D.B., Pulczinski, J.C., Eugene, N. and Satariano, W.A., 2014. Cancer prevention among adults aged 45–64 years: setting the stage. American journal of preventive medicine, 46(3), pp.S1-S6.

Pascual, T., Perrone, G., Morales, S., de la Haba, J., González-Rivera, M., Galván, P., Zalfa, F., Amato, M., Gonzalez, L., Prats, M. and Rojo, F., 2017. Limitations in predicting PAM50 intrinsic subtype and risk of relapse score with Ki67 in estrogen receptor-positive HER2-negative breast cancer. Oncotarget, 8(13), p.21930.

Rosner, B., Eliassen, A.H., Toriola, A.T., Chen, W.Y., Hankinson, S.E., Willett, W.C., Berkey, C.S. and Colditz, G.A., 2017. Weight and weight changes in early adulthood and later breast cancer risk. International journal of cancer, 140(9), pp.2003-2014.

Torre, L.A., Bray, F., Siegel, R.L., Ferlay, J., Lortet-Tieulent, J. and Jemal, A., 2015. Global cancer statistics, 2012. CA: a cancer journal for clinicians, 65(2), pp.87-108.

Webber, C., Jiang, L., Grunfeld, E. and Groome, P.A., 2017. Identifying predictors of delayed

diagnoses in symptomatic breast cancer: a scoping review. European journal of cancer care,

26(2).

White, M.C., Holman, D.M., Boehm, J.E., Peipins, L.A., Grossman, M. and Henley, S.J., 2014.

Age and cancer risk: a potentially modifiable relationship. American journal of preventive

medicine, 46(3), pp.S7-S15.

YOUR KNOWLEDGE HAS VALUE

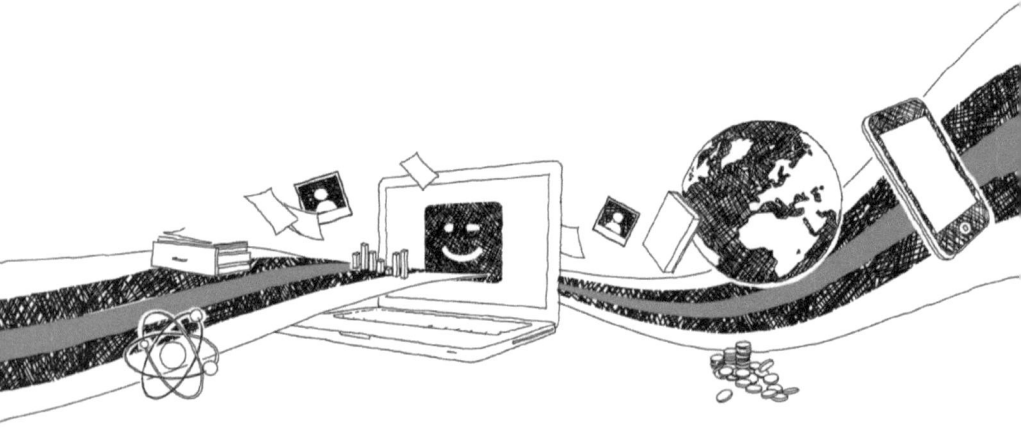

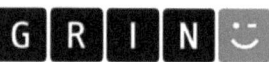